THE TRUTH ABOUT DIETS

WHAT'S RIGHT FOR YOU

OBESITY & KIDS

THE TRUTH ABOUT DIETS

ABOUT DIETS

WHAT'S RIGHT FOR YOU

BY JAMIE HUNT

MASON CREST PUBLISHERS INC.
370 Reed Road
Broomall, Pennsylvania 19008
(866)MCP-BOOK (toll free)
www.masoncrest.com

First Printing
9 8 7 6 5 4 3 2 1

Library of Congress Cataloging-in-Publication Data

Hunt, Jamie.
  The truth about diets : what's right for you? / by Jamie Hunt.
      p. cm.
  Includes bibliographical references and index.
  ISBN 978-1-4222-1710-8 (hardcover)   ISBN 978-1-4222-1705-4 (series)
  ISBN 978-1-4222-1898-3 (pbk.)   ISBN 978-1-4222-1893-8 (pbk. series)
  1. Reducing diets—Juvenile literature. I. Title.
  RM222.2.H857 2010
  613.2'5—dc22

2010010014

Design by MK Bassett-Harvey and Wendy Arakawa.
Produced by Harding House Publishing Service, Inc.
www.hardinghousepages.com
Cover design by Torque Advertising and Design.
Printed in USA by Bang Printing.

CONTENTS

INTRODUCTION FOR THE TEACHERS

We as a society often reserve our harshest criticism for those conditions we understand the least. Such is the case for obesity. Obesity is a chronic and often-fatal disease that accounts for 400,000 deaths each year. It is second only to smoking as a cause of premature death in the United States. People suffering from obesity need understanding, support, and medical assistance. Yet what they often receive is scorn.

Today, children are the fastest growing segment of the obese population in the United States. This constitutes a public health crisis of enormous proportions. Living with childhood obesity affects self-esteem, which down the road can affect employment and attainment of higher education. But childhood obesity is much more than a social stigma. It has serious health consequences.

Childhood obesity increases the risk for poor health in adulthood—but also even during childhood. Depression, diabetes, asthma, gallstones, orthopedic diseases, and other obesity-related conditions are all on the rise in children. Recent estimates suggest that 30 to 50 percent of children born in 2000 will develop type 2 diabetes mellitus, a leading cause of preventable blindness, kidney failure, heart disease, stroke, and amputations. Obesity is undoubtedly the most pressing nutritional disorder among young people today.

If we are to reverse obesity's current trend, there must be family, community, and national objectives promoting healthy eating and exercise. As a nation, we must demand broad-based public-health initiatives to limit TV watching, curtail junk food advertising toward children, and promote physical activity. More than rhetoric, these need to be our rallying cry. Anything short of this will eventually fail, and within our lifetime obesity will become the leading cause of death in the United States if not in the world. This series is an excellent first step in battling the obesity crisis by educating young children about the risks, the realities, and what they can do to build healthy lifestyles right now.

CHAPTER 1
AN OVERWEIGHT WORLD

Did you know that people all over the globe are getting fatter? There are more than 1 billion adults around the world who are **overweight**. At least 300 million of them are **obese**.

But it's not just grownups who are overweight and obese. More and more children are overweight too, even very

DIET MATH

Doctors say you are obese or overweight based on a number called your BMI (body mass index). You can figure out your BMI for yourself.

Take your weight in pounds (or kilograms) and divide it by your height in inches (or meters) squared and then multiply by 703. This means that if you're 4 feet and 7 inches tall (55 inches) and you weigh 75 pounds, the equation will look like this:

$$[75 \div (55 \times 55)] \times 703 =$$
$$(75 \div 3{,}025) \times 703 =$$
$$.025 \times 703 = 17.6$$

According to the U.S. Centers for Disease Control and Prevention, if your BMI is:

below 18.5, you are underweight. (So if your BMI is 17.6, you may be too thin!)
between 18.5 and 25.9, you are normal weight.
between 25.0 and 29.9, you are overweight.
at 30.0 or higher, you are obese.

young children. Around the world, at least 42 million children under five are overweight.

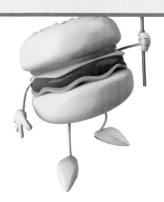

What's the difference between being overweight and being obese? Both words mean that a person has too much body fat, so much so that it's a health risk. But a person who is obese has much more fat than a person who is overweight, and the health risks are greater as well.

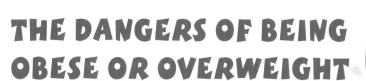

THE DANGERS OF BEING OBESE OR OVERWEIGHT

So what's so bad about being overweight or obese? People come in all different sizes and shapes—and no one should ever be insulted or treated with less respect because of

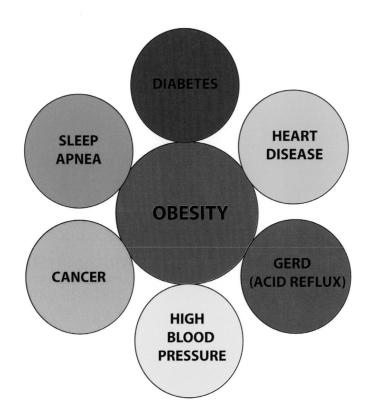

Being overweight or obese increases the chances of many different medical problems.

DID YOU KNOW?

Even though doctors use BMI to determine if you're overweight or obese, BMI is sometimes wrong. That's because people who have lots of muscle can also weigh more, even though they don't have much fat.

their weight. People who are overweight or obese can still be smart and pretty and funny. But being overweight can be dangerous. It puts you at risk for getting sick, both now, when you're still a kid, and later, when you grow up.

Children who are overweight or obese are more likely to get diabetes. This is a disease where your body doesn't break down sugar the way it should. If you have diabetes, you will probably have to take medicine or have special shots every day to help your body process sugar normally. Diabetes can lead to other diseases as well, including blindness. It can make it hard for you to heal after a cut or injury.

Being overweight also increases your chances of having heart disease. This is an illness weusually connect with older people, but carrying too much weight around is hard on your heart, no matter how old you are. Even worse, the heavier you are, the harder it will probably be for you to run around and exercise. Your heart and lungs need exercise to be healthy. Today, more and more children are obese or overweight—and more and more children are getting heart disease.

Overweight children are also likely to stay that way as they grow up. Being obese or overweight when you are an adult can put you at risk for even more diseases. The extra weight puts strain on your

DID YOU KNOW?

Being overweight and not exercising enough causes one-third of all cancers.

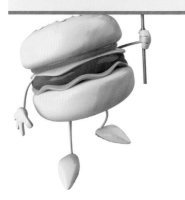

Exercise is important to keep your heart and lungs healthy.

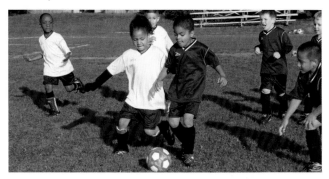

joints, which can lead to arthritis, a disease that makes your joints swollen, stiff, and sore. Obesity may also cause certain kinds of **cancer**.

As people who are overweight or obese grow older, the added weight on their bodies can also lead to other problems, like **high blood pressure** (which increases your chances of having a **stroke**), **gallbladder** disease, and breathing problems. Being overweight can also mean that you have more problems han-

What is cancer? Cancer is a disease that causes the cells in different parts of your body to grow too fast, to the point that they kill healthy cells.

What does high blood pressure and stroke mean? High blood pressure is when blood pushes against the walls of the blood vessels harder than is normal. This tends to happen when the vessels become too narrow.

A stroke is when the cells in your brain suddenly die because they don't get enough blood.

What is your gallbladder? Your gallbladder is an organ in your body that helps you digest fats.

DID YOU KNOW?

At least 2.6 million people each year die as a result of being overweight or obese.

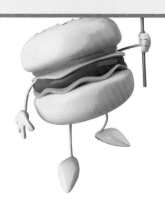

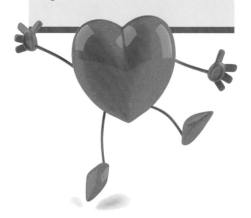

dling your emotions. People who are obese or overweight are more likely to have **depression**.

What is depression?
Depression is an emotional illness that makes people feel very sad most of the time.

Digestive System

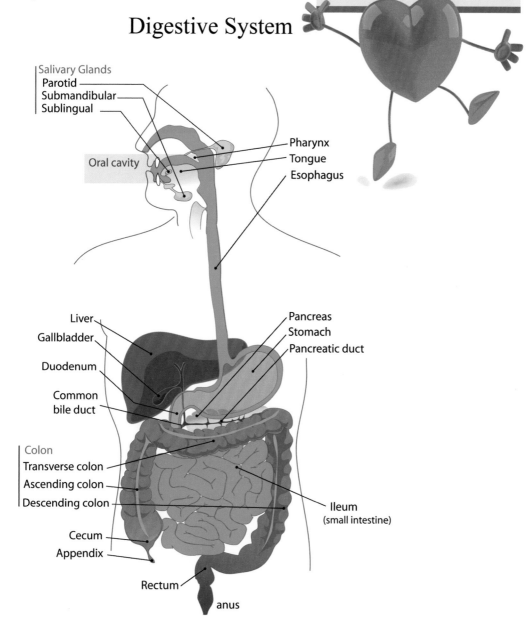

Salivary Glands
Parotid
Submandibular
Sublingual

Oral cavity

Pharynx
Tongue
Esophagus

Liver
Gallbladder
Duodenum
Common bile duct

Pancreas
Stomach
Pancreatic duct

Colon
Transverse colon
Ascending colon
Descending colon

Cecum
Appendix

Ileum
(small intestine)

Rectum
anus

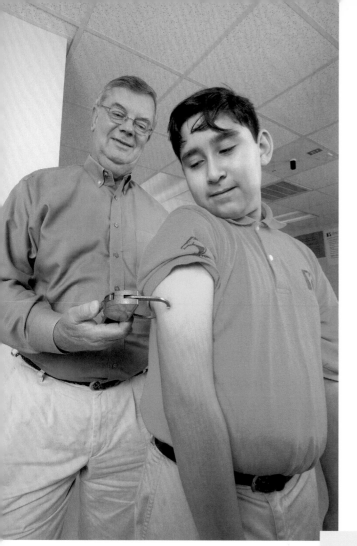

This doctor is using a skin-fold test to learn how much body fat this boy has.

A BIG PROBLEM

There's no denying that obesity is a big problem! It's a problem for individuals who are over-weight or obese—and it's a problem for countries around the world. Dealing with the health prob-lems caused by obesity costs countries millions of dollars. Scientists and doctors are working hard to find the answer to this problem.

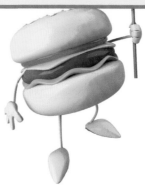

DID YOU KNOW?

Smoking is the number-one cause of deaths that could be prevented. Obesity is the number-two cause of all deaths that could otherwise have been prevented.

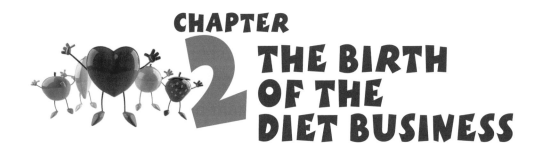

CHAPTER 2
THE BIRTH OF THE DIET BUSINESS

Back in the 1800s, the main things that caused people to get sick or die were **infectious** diseases. People were more likely to catch these diseases if they didn't have a nutritious diet, so doctors and health officials encouraged people to eat *more* of all kinds of food. Doctors even told their patients to gain weight in order to be healthier!

Back in the 19th century, people who had round, plump bodies were considered to be not only healthier, but also wealthier, more upper class. Men thought women with

People have not always thought super-thin women were beautiful—a woman with a more rounded figure was considered the ideal beauty in the 19th century.

What does infectious mean? It means that a disease can spread from one person to another, passed along by viruses or bacteria.

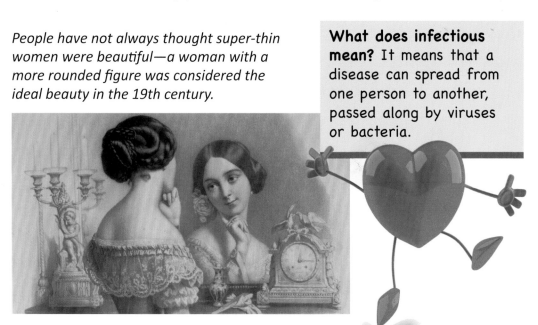

chubby cheeks and dimpled arms were prettier than thin women. People who were very thin were considered to be poor and low class.

A CHANGING OUTLOOK

As the 1800s went past, however, the world changed. New machines of all sorts were being invented, and many of these machines helped grow food, package it, and move it from place to place much more cheaply and quickly. This meant that you no longer had to be rich in order to have plenty of food.

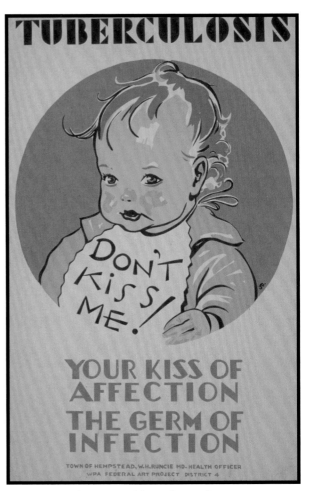

Infectious diseases, like tuberculosis, were a health concern in the 19th century. Poor diet made people more likely to get sick, so eating more and gaining weight were the healthy thing to do.

By the 1920s, upper-class people considered thinness to be a sign of beauty and wealth. Women who had hollow cheeks and bony hips were now considered to be the prettiest.

No one wanted to be fat anymore, and doctors were now advising their patients to lose weight.

But food was plentiful in many parts of the world, and people were still gaining weight. What could they do?

Well, they could go on a diet.

THE BIRTH OF A NEW INDUSTRY

As a result, a new business was born—the diet **industry**. These are the businesses that make diet pills, special low-calorie foods and drinks, and other products intended to help you lose weight. These businesses also include publishers and magazines that sell books and articles about losing weight. Authors and doctors who write about and **specialize** in weight-loss are also a part of this business.

People who are obese need to lose weight, so these businesses and individuals are offering a service people need. These

What does the word industry mean? The way it's used here, where we're talking about the diet industry, it means all the people and companies who are making money by doing a particular thing.

What does it mean to specialize? It means to focus on just one area or thing, so that you become very good at it.

businesses are also getting rich. Today there are thousands of weight-loss products for sale. Everywhere you turn—in magazines, on television, and on billboards—you run into ads for something that is guaranteed to help you lose weight.

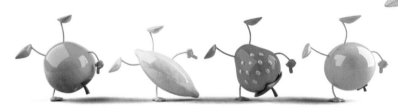

If your scale tells says you are overweight, the diet industry will be ready with suggestions for how to lose weight.

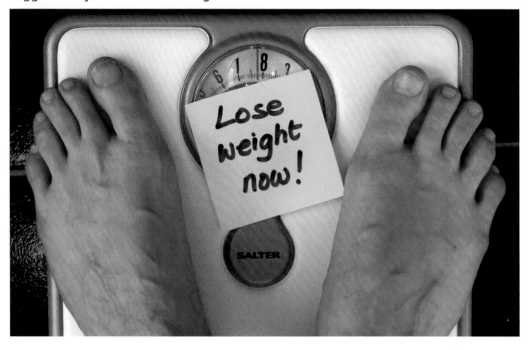

ADVERTISING

When you hear a message often enough, you start to believe it. That's how advertising works. It bombards us with messages, telling us that we NEED to buy a certain thing. Whether it's a car, a pair of jeans, a cell phone, a cleaning product, or a diet product, the ads and commercials are designed to make us want that thing—so that we'll go out and spend our money on it.

THE MEDIA AND BODY SHAPE

The media—newspapers, magazines, radio, television, and the Internet—is full of messages that thin is beautiful. Many people, especially women and girls, have become convinced that they are overweight, even when they're not.

Healthy bodies come in many shapes. Some are small and slender, but others are naturally larger. That doesn't mean the person is overweight. But because the

DID YOU KNOW?

When people who are not overweight believe they need to lose weight, sometimes they end up with an eating disorder. People who have eating disorders may refuse to eat almost anything at all, to the point that they get sick. Or they may eat and eat and eat and eat—and then make themselves throw up or go the bathroom to get rid of all the food before it can make them fat. Either kind of eating disorder can be dangerous. Eating disorders are very serious conditions that can make people very sick. In the United States, more than 7 million women and 1 million men have an eating disorder.

models and actresses we see in magazines, on television, and in movies tend to be super-thin, many of us have become convinced that we all have to look like them in order to be pretty. The reality is, though, that many models are *underweight*. They're *too* thin.

DID YOU KNOW?

People spend billions of dollars on diet foods. In 2005, in the United States alone, people bought $2.4 billion of prepackaged weight-loss meals (like Lean Cuisine© and NutriSystem©), another $1.7 million on shakes and snacks (like SlimFast© and the Zone©), and $15 billion on diet soda.

By the end of the 20th century, everywhere people turned there were messages telling them they needed to be thin. The media was filled with messages that you needed to be skinny in order to be happy or pretty or respected. People became convinced that if they lost weight, they'd not only look better but they'd be happier too. Other people would like them more. Most people thought more about those reasons for losing weight than they did about their health.

No wonder then that people started looking for a "magic answer," the perfect diet plan to help them lose the weight they needed. So when they heard about the latest weight-loss product, they bought it (whether they need to lose weight or not). But many of these weight-loss products didn't keep their promises.

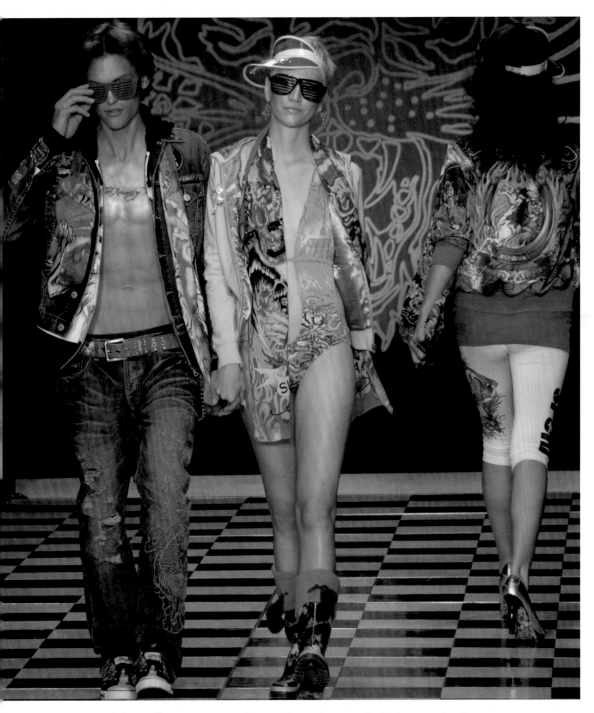

Models walk runways and pose for ads to sell clothes and other products. They also "sell" an unrealistic ideal of thinness.

CHAPTER
3 DIET PLANS

When people want to lose weight, they go on a diet. But what does that really mean?

CALORIES

You've probably heard people talk about calories. Sometimes it may sound as though calories are bad things. After all, commercials are always making low-calorie foods sound as though they're healthier, and people who are on a diet will often count calories. It's true that too many calories can make us fat—but we also need calories.

Calories are a way to measure what's in the food we eat. We use inches and feet (or centimeters and meters) to measure how long or tall something is; we use pints and quarts (or liters) to measure liquids like milk and soda—and we use calories to measure how much **energy** is in a certain food.

What is energy?
Energy is the ability to be active, the power it takes to move your body.

Each one of us needs a certain amount of calories every day to be healthy and have the energy we need for all the things we do in a day. Even sitting still takes a certain number of calories, but the more active we are, the more calories we need. People who are bigger, more active, or who are growing usually need more calories than smaller people, people who don't move around very much, and people who aren't growing.

When we eat more calories than we need, our bodies store the extra energy as fat. Long ago, our ancestors went through times when they had plenty of food, followed by times when food was scarcer. Their bodies' stores of fat helped them get through the times when they had less food. Today, though, many times our bodies just keep storing more and more fat that never needs to be used. When that happens, we end up being over-weight or obese.

Recommended Daily Calories		
Age	Boys	Girls
2	1000	1000
3	1000–1400	1000–1200
4–5	1200–1400	1200–1400
6	1400–1600	1200–1400
7	1400–1600	1200–1600
8	1400–1600	1400–1600
9	1600–1800	1400–1600
10	1600–1800	1400–1800
11	1800–2000	1600–1800
12	1800–2200	1600–2000
13	2000–2200	1600–2000
14	2000–2400	1800–2000
15	2200–2600	1800–2000
16–18	2400–2800	1800–2000
19–20	2600–2800	2000–2200

The amount of calories you need depends on your age, sex and activity level. An active boy or girl needs more calories than a boy or girl of the same age who is less active.

To get rid of these extra stores of fat, we need to do one of two things: take in fewer calories, forcing our bodies to use up the stored energy in our fat—or use up more calories by exercising more, which will also make our bodies use up the fat we've stored.

MANY DIFFERENT PLANS

Losing weight isn't easy. It means you have to change your habits. You have to eat differently—and eating is something most people enjoy! So book publishers and magazines started selling diet plans. Each one was a little different. Some diets said you should eat only one kind of food, other diets said you should eat mostly a different kind of food. Drug companies started making diet pills that were supposed to help people lose weight. (Some of them worked, some of them didn't. The ones that did work

What are side effects? They're something that happens when you take a medicine besides the helpful result you were looking for. For instance, some medicines can cause headaches or stomachaches along with doing something that's good for you. Some side effects aren't very serious, but others can be so dangerous that you shouldn't take that particular medicine.

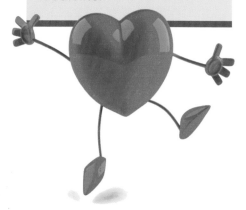

often had dangerous **side effects**.) And all these different kinds of businesses made ads and commercials about their products to convince people that they needed help to lose weight.

These days, there are literally hundreds, if not thousands, of diets out there. If you do a Google search for "diet plan," you'll get nearly 18 million sites to choose from! Some diets have you count calories, some have you count "points." Other diets have you count grams of fat or **carbohydrates**. There are juice diets and grapefruit diets and cabbage soup diets. Some companies sell prepackaged diet foods. Other diet books tell you to eat spoonfuls of olive oil every day—or a big breakfast—or lots of fat.

What are carbohydrates?
Carbohydrates are found in starchy foods like bread, pasta, rice, cereal, and potatoes. They're also found in sugary foods like candy, cookies, and cake. Your body needs carbohydrates every day to get the energy it needs, but some carbohydrates are better for you than others. When you eat too many carbohydrates, the energy from the food gets stored in your body as fat.

Some dieters eat grapefruit with every meal because they think it "magically" burns extra calories.

There is no "quick fix" to lose weight, but that doesn't stop people from trying the next new diet!

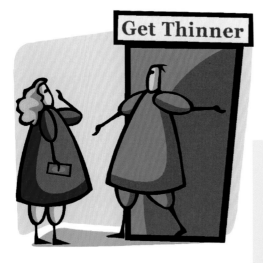

It's confusing! Most diets do work for a while, because almost any diet you follow will mean that you take in fewer calories than you use. But because most diets are

hard work, people don't stick to them—and this means they either don't lose weight or they gain back any weight they lost. When that happens, it's only normal for people to feel discouraged and frustrated.

Then the next thing they know, they see another diet being advertised. "Maybe THIS is the one that will work for me," they say to themselves. And then they buy another magazine or book or diet pill, or they sign up for another diet program.

Grownups make this mistake all the time, but so do teenagers and kids. If there were one diet that worked, all the time, anyone who was overweight would go on that diet, lose weight, and never need to go on a diet again. But that's not the way it works. **Researchers** tell us that 95 percent of all people who lose weight on a diet will gain it back within five years—and some gain back more than they lost, so they end up weighing more than they did when they began.

Calories provide fuel for your body. Eat too little and you will not have enough energy, but overfill your tank and your body will have other health problems.

What are researchers? They're people who study things closely to find out new answers.

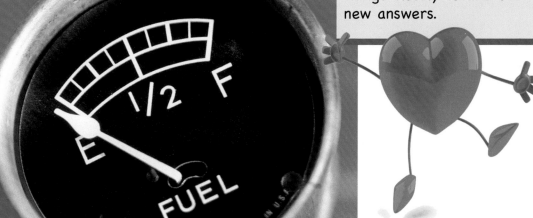

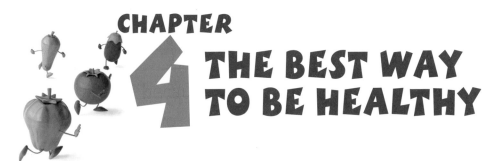

CHAPTER 4
THE BEST WAY TO BE HEALTHY

Experts say that dieting really isn't the best way to lose weight. People may lose weight on a diet, but after a while, most people start feeling frustrated—and HUNGRY! Sooner or later, they go back to eating the way they did before. Sometimes they eat even more than they did before.

The best way to lose weight and be healthy is to change the way you think about food. The first step is to understand what your body really needs to be healthy.

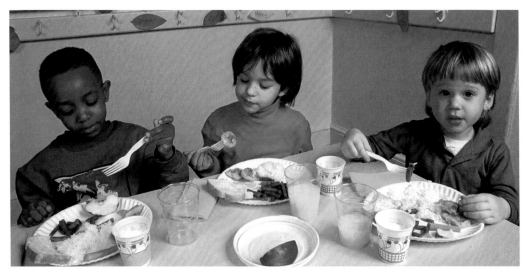

Your body needs food to stay healthy and strong. The key to a healthy weight is learning what foods are the right foods.

GOOD NUTRITION

All foods have calories, whether it's cookies or carrots, lettuce or ice cream, but some foods have more calories than others. This means that if you ate a pound of lettuce, you would have eaten only about 80 calories (and you would have had to eat about 16 cups of lettuce)—but if you ate a pound of chocolate chip cookies (about 10 cookies), you would have eaten 2100 calories! That's a big difference.

Every day, your body needs **nutrition** from many kinds of foods. Different kinds of food contain different **nutrients**, and you need a balanced diet of all of them. That's why any diet plan that tells you to eat mostly one thing—or not at all of another thing— is probably not a very healthy way to eat. Your body needs carbohydrates, fats,

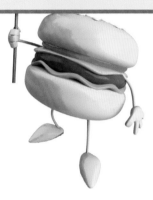

DID YOU KNOW?

An athlete like a bicyclist who is in training for a big race may need to eat as many as 6,000 calories a day.

What does nutrition and nutrients mean?
Nutrition is the process by which your body gets what it needs to live and grow from the food you eat. Nutrients are the things in food that help your body live and grow.

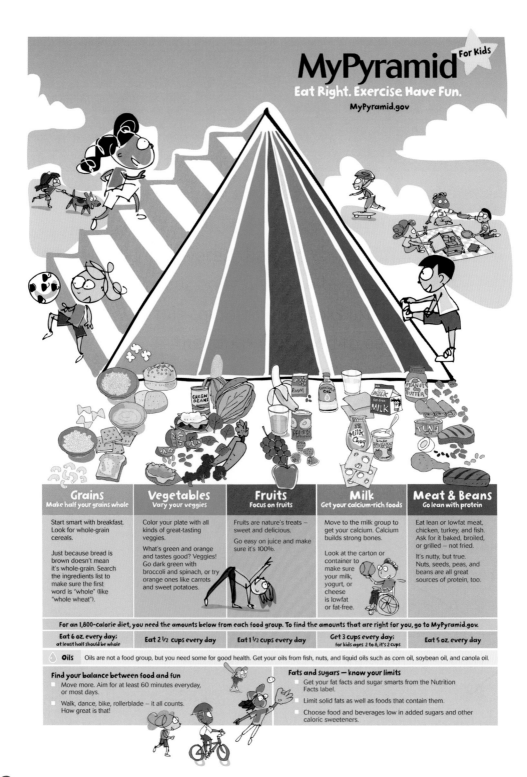

protein, and minerals and vitamins every day. The only way to get what you need of these nutrients, is to eat lots of different kinds of healthy foods.

CARBOHYDRATES

Carbohydrates, found in foods such as grain products, fruits, vegetables, and candy, are important sources of energy for your body. You need to get about 45 to 65 percent of your daily calories from carbohydrates.

Not all carbohydrates, however, are the same, and some are much better for you than others. The healthiest carbohydrates are complex carbohydrates. They are found in whole-grain foods like whole-wheat bread, long-grain brown rice, and oatmeal, and in many vegetables and fruits. Complex carbohydrates take a long time for your body to break down, so they give you energy for a longer period of time. Complex carbohydrates are also important because they are good sources of other nutrients, like vitamins and minerals, as well as fiber.

DID YOU KNOW?

Most children between the ages of 5 and 12 need between 1,200 and 2,000 calories a day. Exactly how much they need will depend on how active they are, whether they're in the midst of a growth spurt, and how big they are.

While you should eat lots of complex carbohydrates, you should eat only a few simple carbohydrates—like sugar, candy, white bread, white rice, and most desserts. Instead of being broken down slowly inside your body, simple carbohydrates break down all at once, flooding your bloodstream with sugar. Usually, your body can't burn this flood of sugar fast enough, so it stores the excess sugar as fat. What's more, many simple carbohydrate foods are packed with calories, but they have very little fiber or other nutrients. That's why they're sometimes called "junk food"—they have lots of "empty" calories, stuff that makes you fat without

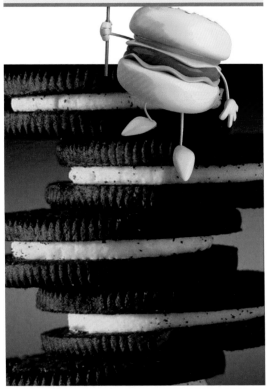

Simple carbohydrates, like the sugar in cookies, should only be eaten in small amounts.

giving you much of the things your body really needs to be healthy.

FATS

Fats have lots of energy. They've gotten a bad reputation, because people think that if you eat fats, you'll *be* fat. But your body needs certain types of fats to be healthy.

Researchers have found that you need to get about 20 to 35 percent of your calories from fats. Each gram of fat you eat has nine calories. That's more than twice the amount of energy contained in a gram of carbohydrates or proteins, so it takes far fewer grams of fat to give you a lot of calories. That's one reason why eating too many fats can make you gain weight.

DIET MATH

To figure out how many grams of carbohydrates you should eat each day, multiply the number of calories you need by .45. Divide the answer by four (the number of calories in a gram of carbohydrate). This gives you the low-end of your necessary carbohydrate intake. Now multiply the number of calories by .65, and divide the answer by four. This gives you the high-end for your carbohydrate intake. Here is an example for a person who needs 2,200 calories each day:

(2200 calories x .45) ÷ 4 calories per gram of carbohydrates = 247.5 grams
(2200 calories x .65) ÷ 4 calories per gram of carbohydrates = 357.5 grams

A person who requires 2,200 calories should eat approximately 247.5 to 357.5 grams of carbohydrates (mostly complex) every day.

So how can you eat fats in a healthy and responsible way? First, you need to know what type of fat you're eating. The three most important categories of fats are unsaturated, saturated, and trans fat. Unsaturated fats are liquid at room temperature. Common examples are olive and vegetable oils. Saturated fats are solid at room temperature. Butter is an example of a saturated fat. Trans fats are unsaturated fats that have undergone a chemical process called hydrogenation to make them solid at room temperature. Margarine and vegetable shortening are the most common trans fats.

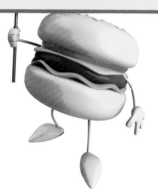

DID YOU KNOW?

Fat is an important part of many body tissues. Your brain and nerves also need fat in order to work the way they should. And fat helps carry certain mportant vitamins to all the parts of your body.

Of these three fat categories, one is safe and two are not. The key to which is which is cholesterol. You cells and nerve tissue need cholesterol to be healthy—but too much cholesterol can be dangerous. Your body produces its own cholesterol, so when you eat too much of it, the extra can build up inside your blood vessels. Eventually, this can block the vessels, which can cause a heart attack or a stroke.

Just as there are "bad" and "good" fats, there are also "bad" and "good" cholesterol. The "bad" cholesterol is called "low-density lipoproteins" (LDL). This is the type of choles-terol that can clog your blood vessels. "High density lipopro-teins" (HDL)—the "good" cholesterol—helps flush LDL choles-terol out of your body. If you have too much LDL cholesterol and not enough HDL cholesterol to get rid of it, your heart and blood vessels can become unhealthy. That's why a fat is considered "bad" or "good" depending on the type of choles-terol it contains.

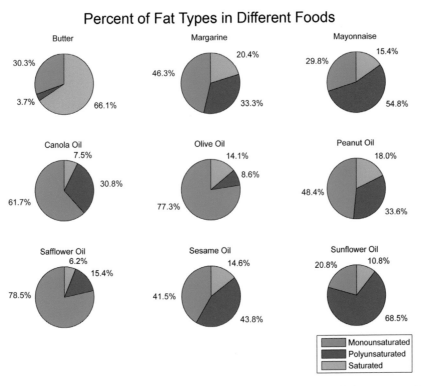

Fats are complicated—your body needs them, but too much of the wrong kind is unhealthy.

What does moderation mean? It means not too much, not too little.

Saturated fats come mostly from animals. They should be eaten in **moderation** because they contain cholesterol and will increase the amount of LDL cholesterol in your blood. You should eat no more than 20 to 25 grams of saturated fat each day, and the less you eat the better.

You can increase your levels of good cholesterol (HDL) by eating certain unsaturated fats. Unsaturated fats come in two forms, monounsaturated and polyunsaturated. Foods like avocados and olive oil are high in monounsaturated fats, while foods like some grains, nuts, and fish

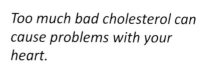

Too much bad cholesterol can cause problems with your heart.

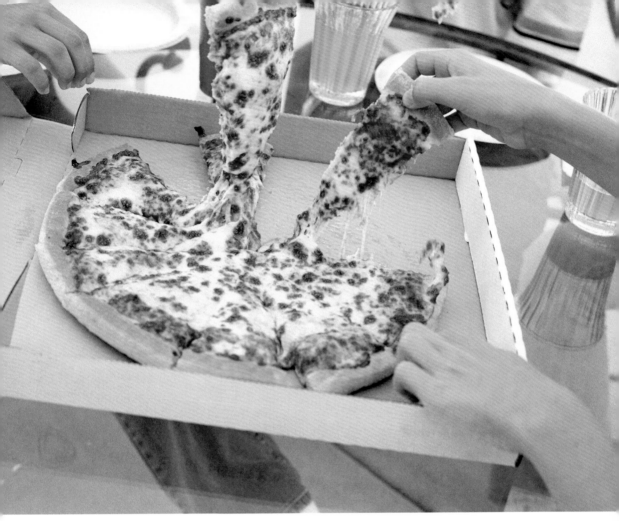

Too much saturated fat is unhealthy, so don't eat too much pizza!

are high in polyunsaturated fats. Polyunsaturated fats, especially those found in certain fish like salmon, lake trout, tuna, and mackerel, contain a lot of HDL cholesterol. Even though unsaturated fats are good for you, however, don't eat too much of them! They have lots of calories, which could make you gain weight.

Scientists today believe that trans fat is the worst kind of fat. Trans fats make LDL cholesterol build up in your body, and your body has a hard time breaking them down. Trans fats are found in snack foods—like crackers, cookies, and other desserts—that contain hydrogenated or partially hydrogenated vegetable oils.

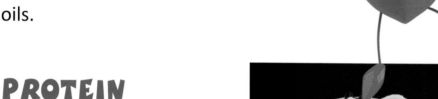

What are dairy products and legumes? Dairy products are any food that contains milk (like cheese, yogurt, and ice cream). Legumes are foods that grow in pods (like beans, lentils, and peas).

PROTEIN

Protein is found in meat, eggs, and **dairy products**, as well as most grains, nuts, and **legumes**. Protein is one of your body's most important building blocks. Without it,

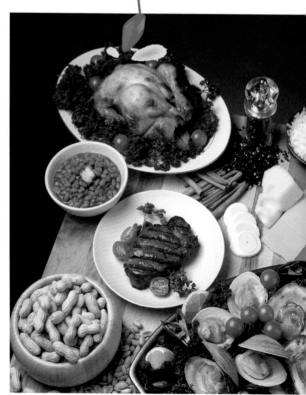

All these foods are a good source of protein.

MORE DIET MATH

To find out how much protein you need each day, multiply the number of calories you need by .10. Divide the answer by four (the number of calories in one gram of protein). This gives you the low-end of your necessary protein intake. Now multiply your calories by .35 and divide by four. This answer gives you the high-end for your protein intake. Here is an example for a person who needs 2,200 calories each day:

(2200 calories x .10) ÷ 4 calories per gram of protein = 55 grams
(2200 calories x .35) ÷ 4 calories per gram of protein = 192.5 grams

A person who needs 2,200 calories each day should eat approximately 55 to 192.5 grams of protein.

What do we mean when we talk about body tissues? Tissues in your body are a group of cells that are alike and that work together to do the same job inside your body.

you could not build or repair your muscles and other body **tissues**. Protein also provides you with calories. You need to get 10 to 35 percent of your daily calories from protein.

VITAMINS AND MINERALS

You also need vitamins and minerals to make your body workthe way it should. Vitamins and minerals are often found in fruit and vegetables.

There are two kinds of vitamins—fat soluble and water soluble. The fat-soluble vitamins—A, D, E, and K—dissolve in fat and can be stored in your body. The water-soluble vitamins—C and the B vitamins (such as vitamins B6, B12, niacin, riboflavin, and folate)—need to be dissolved in water before your body can absorb them. Because of this, your body can't store these vitamins, so any vitamin C or B your body doesn't use leaves your body every day in your urine. That's why you need to eat a fresh supply of these vitamins every day.

Plants and animals make vitamins, but minerals come from the soil and water, and they are then absorbed by plants through their roots or eaten by animals.

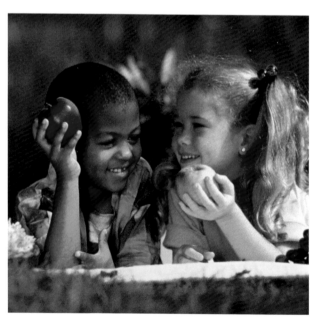

An apple a day may not keep the doctor away, but it will help replace some important water-soluble vitamins.

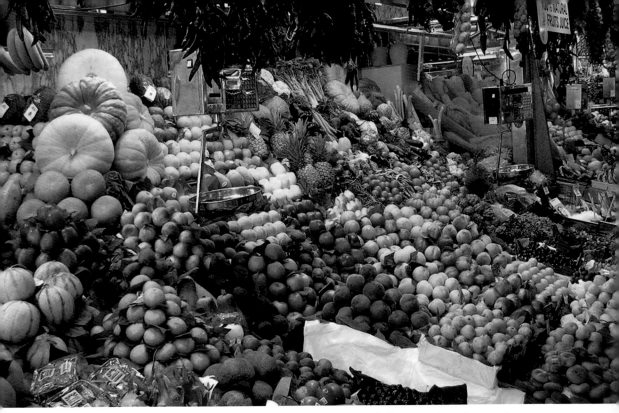

Fruits and vegetables are a colorful way to get many different vitamins and minerals.

Your body needs larger amounts of some minerals, such as calcium (found in dairy products and green leafy vegetables), to grow and stay healthy. Other minerals like chromium, copper, iodine, iron, selenium, and zinc are called trace minerals because you only need very small amounts of them each day.

Vitamins and minerals help you fight off germs and other things that might make you sick. Vitamins and minerals also help you grow, and they help all your cells and organs do their jobs.

A BALANCED DIET

Eating a variety of foods is the best way to get all the vitamins and minerals you need each day, as well as the right balance of carbohydrates, proteins, fats, and calories. Whole or unprocessed foods—foods that are as close as possible to the way they grew naturally, without being frozen, canned, or packaged—are the best choices for getting the nutrients your body needs to stay healthy and grow properly.

Here are some tips for choosing a healthy variety of foods.

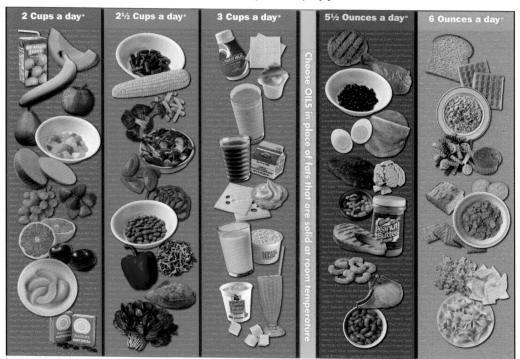

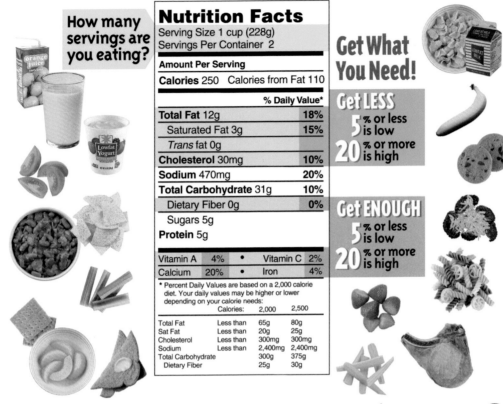

How many servings are you eating?

Nutrition Facts

Serving Size 1 cup (228g)
Servings Per Container 2

Amount Per Serving

Calories 250   Calories from Fat 110

	% Daily Value*
Total Fat 12g	**18%**
Saturated Fat 3g	**15%**
Trans fat 0g	
Cholesterol 30mg	**10%**
Sodium 470mg	**20%**
Total Carbohydrate 31g	**10%**
Dietary Fiber 0g	**0%**
Sugars 5g	
Protein 5g	

Vitamin A	4%	•	Vitamin C	2%
Calcium	20%	•	Iron	4%

* Percent Daily Values are based on a 2,000 calorie diet. Your daily values may be higher or lower depending on your calorie needs:

		Calories:	2,000	2,500
Total Fat	Less than		65g	80g
Sat Fat	Less than		20g	25g
Cholesterol	Less than		300mg	300mg
Sodium	Less than		2,400mg	2,400mg
Total Carbohydrate			300g	375g
Dietary Fiber			25g	30g

Get What You Need!

Get LESS

5 % or less is low

20 % or more is high

Get ENOUGH

5 % or less is low

20 % or more is high

What's the Best Choice for You?

Use the Nutrition Facts Label to Make Choices

Nutrition labels are a great source of information about the food you are eating. Use them to make healthy diet choices.

Does this mean you have to give up foods like potato chips, candy bars, and cookies forever? No, it's okay to have these foods once in a while. Just don't eat too many of them. To choose healthier foods, check food labels, and then pick foods that are high in vitamins and minerals. For example, if you're choosing a drink, a glass of milk is a good source of vitamin D, calcium, phosphorous, and potassium, but a glass of soda has very few vitamins or minerals, if any—but it does have lots of calories!

The best way to lose weight, experts tell us, is to change the way you live. Don't try to make your body do without the things it needs, and don't worry about making yourself look like a skinny actor or actress you've seen on television. Instead, learn to take care of your body. Feed it when it's hungry. Give it the foods it needs to be healthy. Find fun ways to get more exercise, which will also help keep your body at the right weight. Get plenty of sleep.

Do what's best for you!

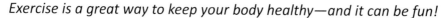

Exercise is a great way to keep your body healthy—and it can be fun!

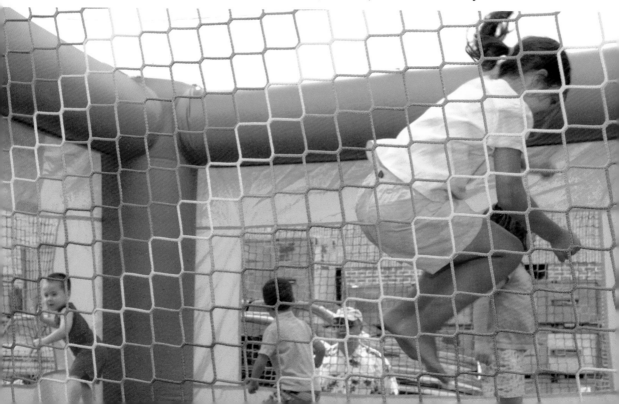

READ MORE ABOUT IT

Bean, Anita. *Awesome Foods for Active Kids: The ABCs of Eating for Energy and Health*. Alameda, Calif.: Hunter House, 2006.

Berg, Frances M. *Children and Teens Afraid to Eat*. Hettinger, N.D.: Healthy Weight Network, 2001.

Dolgoff, Joanna. *Red Light, Green Light, Eat Right: The Food Solution That Lets Kids Be Kids*. Emmaus, Penn.: Rodale, 2009.

Gaesser, Glenn. *Big Fat Lies: The Truth About Your Weight and Your Health*. Carlsbad, Calif.: Gürze Books, 2002.

Lillien, Lisa. *Hungry Girl 1-2-3: The Easiest, Most Delicious, Guilt-Free Recipes on the Planet*. New York: St. Martin's, 2010.

Vos, Miriam B. *The No-Diet Obesity Solution for Kids.* Bethesda, Md.: AGA Institute, 2009.

Zinczenko, David and Matt Goulding. *Eat This Not That! For Kids!* Emmaus, Penn.: Rodale, 2008.

FIND OUT MORE ON THE INTERNET

American Dietetic Association
www.eatright.org

Centers for Disease Control and Prevention
www.cdc.gov

DietFacts
www.dietfacts.com

Diet Information
www.diet-i.com

The Healthy Weight Network
www.healthyweight.net

National Association to Advance Fat Acceptance
www.naafa.org

National Center for Health Statistics
www.cdc.gov/nchs

National Food Laboratory
www.thenfl.com

National Institutes of Health
www.nih.gov

National Library of Medicine
www.nlm.nih.gov

The websites listed on this page were active at the time of publication. The publisher is not responsible for websites that have changed their address or discontinued operation since the date of publication. The publisher will review and update the websites upon each reprint.

INDEX

PICTURE CREDITS

ABOUT THE AUTHOR

Jamie Hunt is a certified teacher who has taught health to children from eleven to thirteen years old. She has worked with many publishers on a number of health-related books for young people. She lives in New York State.